Breast Cancer

The Little Book of Hope

Breast Cancer

The Little Book of Hope

Joyce Giannini, M.A.

GIANNINI PRESS
Los Angeles, CA

Atlas Books
P.O. Box 388
Ashland, OH 44805
Tel: 1 (800) 266-5564
Fax: 1 (419) 281-6883
www.atlasbooks.com
www.breastcancerhopebook.com
joyce@breastcancerhopebook.com

The information contained in this book is intended to be educational and not for diagnostic, prescription, or treatment of any medical disorder whatsoever. The intent of the author is to offer information to help you in your quest for emotional and spiritual well-being. The content of this book is offered as an adjunct to a rational and responsible healthcare program prescribed by a healthcare practitioner. The author is in no way liable for any misuse of the material and assumes no responsibility for your actions.

ISBN 978-0-9798921-0-3
Library of Congress Control Number: 2007906643

First printed in 2008 in the United States of America

Book design by Dotti Albertine (AlbertineBookDesign.com)

Dedication

To my devoted husband and best friend, Ahmad.

To my wonderful mother, Mercedes, my mentor
with forty-three years of survival from breast cancer;
she is and has always been my "bringer of joy".

To my father, the Honorable Peter E. Giannini,
without whom this book never would have come
to fruition. My father's wisdom, love
and support are unsurpassed.

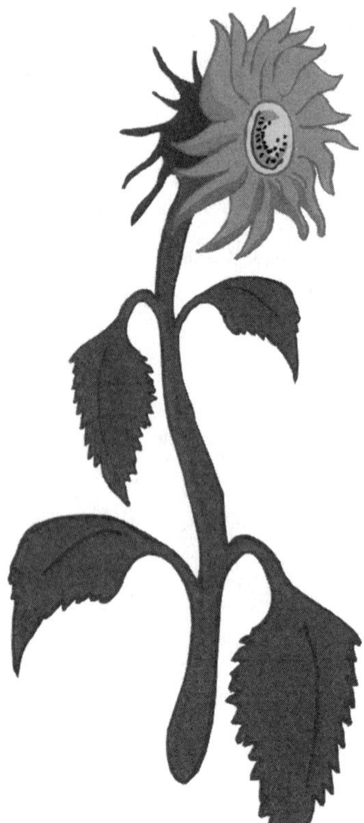

Acknowledgments

I WOULD LIKE TO ACKNOWLEDGE the following people for assisting me in the creation of this book: Dotti Albertine of Albertine Book Design; Bettyanne Bruin of Writers Literary Services, Sheila Zovar of Best Word Processing and Alan Gadney of onebookpro.com for their enthusiasm regarding the publication of this book.

Also, special thanks to Dr. Bret Taback, my breast surgeon; Dr. Linda Li, my reconstructive breast surgeon; my prior oncologist, Dr. Kanchana Anand and my current oncologist, Dr. Lasika Seneviratne.

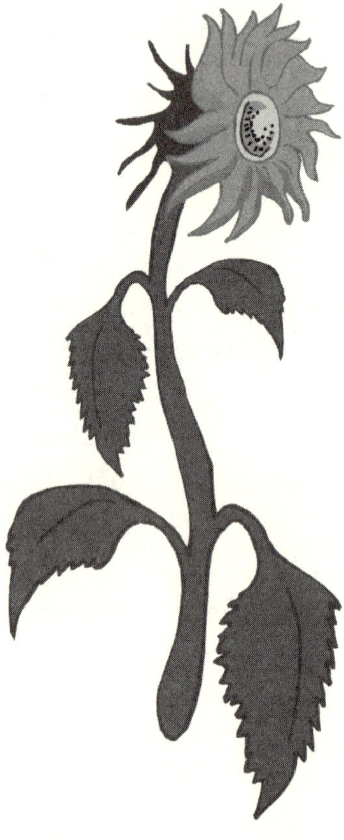

Contents

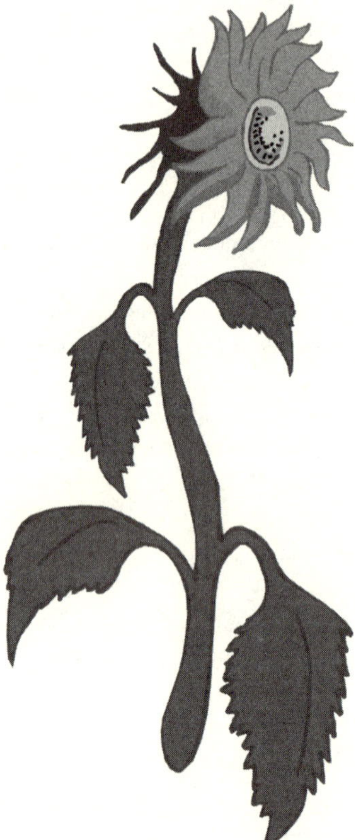

Introduction

YOU FOUND A LUMP OR TWO or maybe even several lumps. It is not the end of the world. In fact, for you it is just the beginning of a journey that will eventually bring you to a happier place with yourself and with your life, if you allow it. I personally have had breast cancer twice in the last five years, and now have a 95 percent chance cure prognosis! At the time of my diagnosis, I was forty-one, single with a boyfriend, Ahmad Jafarbay (my Mongolian Turk), whom I had been dating for one year. We were married two years after my chemo.

When the breast cancer returned in 2004, Ahmad stayed with me through my double mastectomy and implant reconstruction. Some men truly have good hearts. While many men leave their wives or girlfriends if they find out that they have breast cancer, don't worry. If you do the things necessary to take care of yourself you too will be okay. And, like others, you may just meet your true soul mate through this journey.

Ahmad was actually the one who found the first lump in 2001. It was the most aggressive type of Infiltrating Ductal Carcinoma tumor known. Yet, fortunately, the lymph nodes had not been affected. I had a lumpectomy, chemotherapy and radiation. My cancer was estrogen-positive, which meant it was fed by estrogen. I was instructed by my oncologist to take Tamoxifin for five years because this would ensure my entry into menopause. Stubborn as I am, however, I only took the Tamoxifin for about eight months as I was intent upon trying to have a baby. The first thing to learn is, follow your doctor's instructions. So quite surprisingly my cancer returned in October 2004. Since then I have followed, and continue to follow the instructions of my doctors.

Interestingly, according to the *Los Angeles Times Health* January 7, 2007 issue, eighty percent of breast cancer patients have estrogen-specific breast cancer. That means that their breast cancer is fueled by estrogen.

However, according to the article as many as one-third of women stop taking the prescribed aromatose-inhibiting (estrogen-depleting) drugs before the recommended five-year course of therapy, mostly because of the side effects. As I myself experienced, it is very risky to stop taking the aromatose-inhibiting drugs for *any* reason. It is like playing Russian Roulette with your life. It worries doctors who say that women could be reducing their chance of survival. According to my oncologist, because I stopped taking the Tamoxifin after only eight months of compliance, in December 2004 my cancer returned.

Being perplexed, I say,
"Lord, make it right!
Night is as day to
Darkness as light.
I am afraid to touch
Things that involve so much;
My trembling hand may shake,
My skilless hand may break;
Thine can make no mistake."
Being in doubt I say,
"Lord, make it plain;
Which is the true, safe way?

Which would be gain?
I am not wise to know,
Nor sure of foot to go;
What is so clear to Thee,
Lord, make it clear to me!"
—*Streams in the Desert*
by Mrs. Chas E. Cowman

Despite the fact that the doctor had told me I needed only one mastectomy with reconstruction, I decided to have a double mastectomy with reconstructive implants. He said a plastic surgeon could match the breasts. It was quite difficult for me to fathom that a doctor could actually match one breast with the other; however, apparently it is possible. To me, I thought that was something only God could do. I also came to the conclusion that I'd rather not have to worry about the cancer returning in the other breast. And, personally, I wanted to have two perky breasts rather than one that was going north and one that was going south.

I have peace now because I believe, without a doubt that, for whatever reasons, I was not meant to have my own biological baby. So, who knows, maybe one day we will adopt, but not right now. And that is okay, because what happens to us is usually what it was meant to be. Plus, our "baby" is our little Maltese dog, and we are very happy with our little family.

When the cancer returned in 2004 it was on top of my lumpectomy scar. Breast cancer loves to bind onto scars. At the time I was scared that not only might I have to have a mastectomy, but that the lymph nodes could have been affected. I was really terrified that I would once again lose my hair due to chemo!

Thankfully, the second tumor had not spread to the lymph nodes, so hair loss was not an issue. In 2001, after my lumpectomy, chemo and radiation, I had a 73 percent chance of survival for at least five years. Amazingly, however, after the recurrence in 2004, followed by the decision to have a double mastectomy, my doctor told me that I now have a 95 percent chance of survival—as long as I continue to follow his instructions by taking Arimidex, an estrogen blocker, for at least five years. I also get quarterly manual lymph node checks by my oncologist.

We are also very happy with the reconstruction and with how they can actually make the nipples look so natural! It's truly amazing what they can do these days due to the advances in breast cancer research. And it's also truly amazing what God can do for you through this journey, especially at a time when life can seem to be so difficult.

You'll never know the blessings that are there for you to gain if you don't do what it takes to find them. You can get through it, just like the millions of others who are doing so these days. That is what this book is about.

If there's hope for me, there's also hope for you.

In the bitter waves of woe
Beaten and tossed about
By the sullen winds that blow
From the desolate shores of doubt,
Where the anchors that faith has cast
Are dragging in the gale,
I am quietly holding fast
To the things that cannot fail.

And fierce though the fiends may fight,
And long though the angels hide,
I know that truth and right
Have the universe on their side;
And that somewhere beyond the stars
Is a love that is better than fate.
When the night unlocks her bars
I shall see Him—and I will wait.

—Washington Gladden

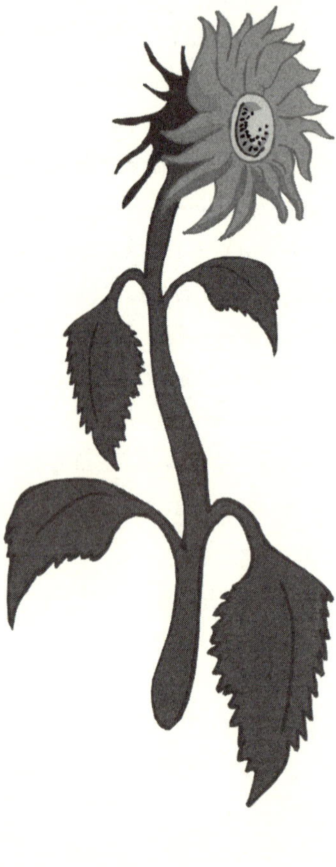

CHAPTER ONE

The Little Pea That Wasn't

It all began in October 2001 when Ahmad and I were quietly watching television. On his own, he casually began doing a breast check. Finding what felt like a little pea-sized "bump" in my right breast, he said, "I don't like this bump."

Of course I said, "What bump?" I felt around, and then grew upset at not being able to find it. Ahmad gently led my hand to a very deep part of my breast, and I felt a small bump about the size of a little pea.

I was forty-one, had never been married and did not have any children, both of which I had longed for my whole life. Men had proposed to me before, but those relationships never felt right except for one, who I now thank God I didn't end up marrying. If he wasn't able to stay faithful to me then, he never would have been after the diagnosis of breast cancer. Ah, no. But the husband God has given me is just what I asked for. He is my best friend and he is my soul mate.

For some reason, however, instead of expressing this gratitude to Ahmad, I became angry with him. "I'm sure it's just a cyst, and you're just being a (bleeping) perfectionist." There I sat, madder than a hatter at him. After a couple of minutes I said, "My insurance won't even kick in for another month, so what am I supposed to do about it?"

"Well, honey," he said, "You've got to get it checked out." I said, "Okay, but I'm just going to have to wait until my insurance kicks in."

"Okay," he said, not wanting to make me afraid that maybe he was onto something that I wasn't. "But I wish you would get it checked sooner."

In all honesty, I said to myself, my mother did have breast cancer when she was forty-three. But still I was sure that mine was nothing more than a cyst…la, la, la, la laaahland….Along I went, happily in denial. I was afraid, but I knew that I had to have insurance if this was breast cancer. So, off I went to work wondering what to do. For as long as I could I continued my daily routine, so that I felt my life was still "normal." I could have a nervous breakdown later.

About three weeks later while my mother and I were having lunch, I began to tell her about the little "pea," and my desire to wait until I had insurance before going in and having this thing checked out. However, she snitched on me that night and told my father. Of course he insisted I get it checked out immediately whether or not I had insurance.

Some of us are not so lucky as to have such loving and supportive parents in our lives. The good news is, though, that even if a person has no money, every state has at least one hospital that is required to perform a mastectomy with reconstruction for free. There are also cancer centers all around the world, willing to guide and help you to all of the resources you need. I truly thank God for my parents, and my job worked things out so that my health insurance kicked in immediately.

So, off I was on the journey that brought me back to God and opened up a sincere appreciation for each day of life. My gratitude for the many blessings that came forth through this most difficult time of my life also grew.

I made an appointment for the next day to have the little pea examined by a gynecologist in Santa Monica, California, which is very near where we live. When the doctor felt the lump he immediately called The Breast Center in Santa Monica. He spoke to a doctor there and ordered an ultrasound and a needle biopsy for the very next day. So, on a Friday in early October 2001, which also happened to be Breast Cancer Awareness month, Ahmad and I were off to get an ultrasound and a needle biopsy.

Ahmad was such a comfort. He held my hand through the entire process. When we saw the large black olive-shaped lump on the ultrasound we both sort of knew what was going on. So did the doctor. The little pea had grown and transformed into a large black olive. The doctor said, "Your left breast looks great! Unfortunately, your right breast doesn't look so good." Then he did the needle biopsy, didn't say a word, and we left.

"Well, honey," I said to Ahmad, "he didn't say it was cancer for sure."

"Yes, honey," Ahmad replied, dousing my hopeful denial, "but the doctor made no indication whatsoever that it was not cancer."

Because the test was taken on a Friday morning I had to wait until Monday for the results. But Ahmad was very reassuring. "It's okay, sweetheart, we'll get through this together, no matter what it is."

Now was he a Godsend or what? Well, I knew that I was in for three very long days.

How to Get Through Those Long Days of Waiting

Trying to keep myself busy, I went back to work that afternoon. In fact, I stayed a little late just to pass the time. I also doubled my Prozac. That night we watched a funny movie. The next morning we cried and prayed together. Then, by myself I went into the bedroom and picked up my dusty Bible and a daily inspirational meditative reading book. I began to read and pray and surrender my results to God. Then I got a manicure and a pedicure.

Later that afternoon, I went to the Wellness Community Cancer Center where I sat among all of the loving people who helped me feel safe in my fear. I browsed through the books on breast cancer in their library and borrowed one of their relaxation tapes. I made an appointment to consult with the group coordinator so I could join a cancer group. Later, I took a bubble bath. Then I listened to the wonderful relaxation tape.

It is very important to talk to someone who knows about the agony of waiting for your breast cancer results. Believe me, when you go to a cancer community group, you will feel right at home. And they are in almost every city and many countries in the world these days. Just ask your local hospital. You'll find out that so many other people are going through just what you are going through, and they will share their stories, their hopes, their fears, and you can bounce your questions off of them and get loving feedback as well as valuable information.

Whatever you do, DO NOT BE ALONE, especially during this waiting time. If you do not have a partner, spend a few nights at a relative or a friend's house. If the local cancer center isn't open, go online or call the American Cancer Society hotline. They are open 24/7 and can be of much comfort to you. If you are able to afford a massage and/or facial, I suggest you go to the spa and hang out there for as many hours as it takes for you to feel serene. Watch funny movies. Walk your dog more often if you have one. Take him or her on different routes to avoid becoming bored. If you catch yourself looking at the cement for more than a couple of minutes, lift up your chin. Look around you and find something you appreciate. Look at the sky and appreciate the sun, the clouds, and all of the wonderful changes of weather.

While waiting, some other suggestions for things to do to pass the time in a relaxing way are:

- Walk on the boardwalk with a friend or two.
- Go window shopping.
- Buy something nice for yourself—maybe some bubble bath, candles, and a new nightgown.
- Take some time to go to your church, temple, mosque, the beach, the meadows, the mountains or wherever you need to go to find God. I went to church and lit a candle for myself, and just prayed and prayed and cried until I received peace in my heart.
- Go online. You will find many breast cancer websites where you can chat with other women, and they can answer your questions or at least give you some comfort. A few good websites you can go to are: www.bcsupport.org, www.breastcancer.org, www.thebreastsite.com, and www.cancer.com.

Monday arrived and the wait actually hadn't been as hard as I had thought since I'd kept myself so busy. With both of my parents on the line I called the doctor, and he explained to me that the biopsy basically came out as a "fibro adenoma with abnormal cells."

I thought, "What in the world does this mean? Is this like being sort-of pregnant?" But of course I didn't ask him this.

Instead, he continued. "Well, both the pathologist and I are still pretty sure it is positive for breast cancer, so we're going to have to do a Core Biopsy."

Now that was a scary term! "What is that?" I asked. "How do you do that?"

"Oh, it's just a procedure that uses a little bigger needle," he said calmly, "and we take some tissue from the core of the tumor." And I was going to have to wait another three days to have this done? Well, I went back to work and kept myself busy, busy, busy.

Mom, Sis and I Have all Been through Breast Cancer and Yet There's No Genetic Link?

Over 211,000 women in the United States are diagnosed with breast cancer each year. Amazingly, approximately 80 percent of the women who get breast cancer are not genetically predisposed to it. I happen to have a strong family history of breast cancer, but we've all made it so far and we all have an excellent chance of recovery! My mother had breast cancer forty-three years ago and is very healthy and happy at age eighty-six today. Within a year after my first diagnosis one of my sisters had a prophylactic, or preventative, double mastectomy where they found Lobular Carcinoma in Situ, a precursor to breast cancer. Today she is healthy and happier for the journey, as well as the spirituality her diagnosis brought into her life.

My sister and I were tested to find out if we were genetically predisposed to breast cancer. We took the BRCA I & II tests, short for Breast Cancer I and Breast Cancer II and we tested negative! My mom said that if we were negative, she obviously was also. She still, however, continues faithfully to receive her annual mammogram.

My Twin Sister Does Not Have Breast Cancer

My twin sister, Sharon, and I are fraternal twins. I was born with dark brown hair and dark brown eyes. She was born with blonde hair and green eyes! So we come from two separate eggs, not one egg that split like identical twins do. That means that our genes are more like natural sisters rather than like identical twins. Sharon has a much lower risk of getting breast cancer than I did. However, according to the national statistics, she still has a 37 percent chance of getting breast cancer (mostly due to family history, dense breasts), which is still quite high. So one day she may get it, but so far she has been able to avoid it.

This is due to several factors. First of all, she started her menstrual cycle a year later than me, which (according to the Risk Factors) is significant because I started producing estrogen at a younger age and therefore I was exposed to estrogen for a longer period of time.

Second, Sharon was married and had her first child at age nineteen. She had her second at age twenty-one. According to the Risk Factors, the earlier a woman has children the lesser the risk of her getting breast cancer. In fact, recent studies have found that having children after age twenty-five raises a woman's probability of getting breast cancer. Third, Sharon has been a vegetarian for at least ten years. I personally believe that the longer a person is a vegetarian, or at least eats organic meat, the more they lessen their chances of getting breast cancer. That will be explained further in another chapter. This is not to say that my twin sister will never get breast cancer; however, I am so happy to know in my own heart that her lifestyle has lessened her odds significantly.

If Someone Leaves You Because of Breast Cancer

Just a little encouragement for those of you whose husband, boyfriend, partner or friend(s) left you because of this disease. You are not alone. An incredible amount of men leave their wives or girlfriends over breast cancer. Now there's true love for you. OUCH! This kind of heartache can only be healed with TIME and the support of others going through the same thing. You may also find that someone you trusted is not who you thought they were. It is amazing how many of us have gone through this only to find that many of our "friends" abandoned us. Interestingly, those whose breast cancer is in a more advanced stage seem to find the most "friends" who abandon them.

Then we find that at least one girlfriend or family member became jealous of us, thinking we just wanted to get free breast enhancements! Well, believe me, one day you'll be glad those people are out of your life because this leaves room for the right people, or person, to enter your life. So—should you find you've lost one of the greatest relationships in your life—just remember you may, in fact, have gained an opportunity to find some of the most beautiful blessings around.

Whether you know it or not, there is Someone out there who sees the bigger picture. In the end, you'll be able to find and get to know your Creator better. You will begin to understand and appreciate the reasons you were given this trial. You'll find an appreciation for life that you can only receive by going through this journey! You'll find some of the most beautiful things life can bring, and that all of these awarenesses are free if you'll just reach outside yourself to find them. You can find true hope and serenity if you let yourself, and if you push yourself to do the things you need to do in order to take care of yourself. Wonderful people can come into your life, if you let them! You may even find your true soul mate. And you'll also get closer than ever to those who really do love you. You'll find friends who will last forever.

Dear restless heart, be still; don't fret and worry so;
God has a thousand ways His love and help to show;
Just trust, and trust, and trust, until His will you know.

Dear restless heart, be still, for peace is God's own smile,
His love can every wrong and sorrow reconcile;
Just love, and love, and love, and calmly wait awhile.

Dear restless heart, be brave; don't moan and sorrow so,
He hath a meaning kind in chilly winds that blow;
Just hope, and hope, and hope, until you braver grow.

Dear restless heart, repose upon His breast this hour,
His grace is strength and life, His love is bloom and flower;
Just rest, and rest, and rest, within His tender power.

Dear restless heart, be still! Don't struggle to be free;
God's life is in your life, from Him you may not flee;
Just pray, and pray, and pray, till you have faith to see.

—Edith Willis Linn

Long-term Vegetarians Have a Significantly Lower Risk of Getting Breast Cancer; Organic Beef is Better for Us

My eldest sister, Christine, has been a vegetarian for her entire adult life and she does not have breast cancer. It is interesting to me that people who have been vegetarians for *most* of their lives have a 40 percent lesser risk of getting breast cancer. It is a known fact that animal fat, especially from red meat and high fat dairy products, especially during the pre-menopausal years, is linked to a higher risk of breast cancer.

There are also other factors to consider regarding breast cancer. There is environmental pollution that can increase our risk. Also, most of the vegetables and fruit we eat have, at some point, been sprayed in the fields with pesticides in order to kill the bugs that might eat them. We might want to consider washing our fruit and vegetables thoroughly or just buying organic. However, nothing compares with the carcinogens in the beef we eat. So if you, like me, enjoy eating a steak or a hamburger once in a while, you might want to think about buying it organic. You also may want to start drinking organic milk, since non-organic cow's milk is tainted with the same carcinogens as the beef. Just something to think about.

What's the Beef?

Cancers of all kinds are escalating in America. Interestingly, China, Japan and India have the lowest rates of breast cancer in the world. Why? Because, compared to the U.S., China and Japan have extremely high standards with regard to the beef they allow into their country. Indians do not eat cattle due to religious reasons. Both China and Japan have had a moratorium on importing U.S. beef because of mad cow disease as well as other reasons.

According to Samuel E. Epstein, M.D., Chairman, Cancer Prevention Coalition, Professor Emeritus Environmental and Occupational Medicine, University of Illinois at Chicago School of Public Health, "U.S. beef is heavily contaminated with sex hormones. When U.S. beef cattle enter feedlots, sex hormone pellets are implanted under the ear skin, a process that is repeated at the midpoint of their 100-day pre-slaughter/fattening period. These hormones increase the weight of the cattle, adding to industry profits by about $80 per animal. Europe, however, has rightly viewed U.S. claims (that the beef is non-carcinogenic) with considerable skepticism and, since 1989, the European Union has banned the sale of beef from hormone-treated cattle."

An unpublicized random USDA survey of thirty-two large feedlots found that as many as half the cattle had illegal, "misplaced implants," in their muscle rather than under the skin of the ear. This "misplacement" can result in very high concentrations of hormone in meat all over the body of the cattle.

Increased levels of sex hormones are linked ever more closely to the escalating increase of reproductive cancers in the U.S.: 37 percent for post-menopausal breast cancer, 46 percent for testicular cancer, and 88 percent for prostate cancer since 1975.

It is widely recognized that American women have about a five-fold greater risk of breast cancer than Japanese women. However, as recently confirmed by studies of cancer rates in Los Angeles County, the most highly populated and ethnically diverse county in the U.S., the low risk factor in Japanese women increases sharply in immigrants to the U.S. after one or two generations." http://newconnexion.net/article/03-06/boycott_beef.html

Alternative Medicine: The Power of the Seedling

There is a particular vitamin in a certain fruit that was the subject of great controversy over thirty-five years ago, when some of the world's top scientists claimed that when this fruit is consumed the vitamin components inside a raw apricot seed made it 100 percent impossible to develop cancer. Further, according to the scientists, Vitamin B17 also known as Laetrile and Amygdalin, will kill existing cancer in most cases. As a preventative, Dr. Krebs, the scientist who discovered the B17 vitamin, strongly claimed that when one eats approximately seven apricot seeds per day (prior to ever getting cancer), they can possibly avoid getting cancer all together.

According to *Cure Magazine's* Spring 2007 issue, "Laetrile, a naturally occurring substance derived primarily from apricot pits, is used by injection, oral tablets, in enemas and topical solutions. Supporters claim cancer cells have more of a certain enzyme in them that splits Laetrile molecules and releases the cyanide within them, thus killing the cancer cells. Another theory claims cancer is a vitamin deficiency that Laetrile can cure." (*Cure Magazine* Spring 2007, p. 29)

Apparently, the pharmaceutical companies did not appreciate this finding.

Pharmaceutical companies only conduct studies on patented chemicals they invent so that, at the end of their study, if the drug gets approved, they have sole rights to its sale. They demanded that the FDA conduct studies on Vitamin B17. In fact, the pharmaceutical companies, in conjunction with the medical establishment, pushed the FDA into making it illegal to sell "raw" apricot seeds or the B17 vitamin with information about its effects on cancer. Because of the raids the FDA made on stores with the apricot containing the B17 vitamin approximately thirty-five years ago, for many years grocery stores did not sell "raw" apricot seeds. Nor did they sell apricots due to the fear of being raided by the FDA.

For several years, we as consumers could not get raw apricots seeds in our grocery stores. We could only buy the sun dried seeds which have all the important enzymes killed off. Now that the B17 apricot topic is no longer a hot topic and has basically been forgotten, we can once again buy apricots in grocery stores.

The book, *World without Cancer* by G. Edward Griffin covers a lot of information on studies that were covered up and talks of great scientists who were arrested when they began telling others about the truth of B17 vitamin. The good news is, for us who already have breast cancer, eating seven apricot seeds per day has proven to significantly shrink tumors. The B17 vitamin found in apricots is also found in other fruits such as apples, peaches, cherries and grapes.

Timing, however, is very important in the use of apricot seedlings. When it comes to using the apricot seedlings, the best results come prior to a person getting chemotherapy. The reason for this is that chemotherapy destroys all living cells, both good and bad, including blood cells. It is well known that in order to assist the blood that has not been damaged you can add extra iron to your diet.

Prior to the making of the Laetrile injections, oral tablets, enemas or topical solutions, according to the experts apricot seeds or any of the other anti-cancer seeds could, and should be chopped up and pulverized because the anti-cancer ingredients are activated in this way. The anti-cancer ingredients in the apricot seed in particular is in the seedlings inside the outer seed. They can be added to food or chopped up and swallowed with a teaspoon of honey or applesauce. Start with a low dosage, as the seed particles must go through your digestive tract and can cause nausea which, if this happens, means you are taking too many seeds too quickly. One or two of the B17 vitamin tablets (100 mg) is an acceptable initial supplemental dosage per day. In nearly all cases when the B17 vitamin is (eventually) taken in high doses, the tumor shrinks.

Interestingly, the study on apricot therapy was conducted at the famous cancer institute, Sloan Kettering, but the study was covered up because of politics. You can find the full explanation of the politics of cancer as well as the results of the Vitamin B17 studies in the book, *World Without Cancer.*

I am neither a doctor nor a nutritionist, so if your doctor recommends that you have chemo and radiation you should follow his or her instructions. I am simply letting you know that there are other options out there to choose from if you do not want to use Western Medicine. To learn more about the phenomenon of the apricot seedlings, you can look at www.1awesomeb17site.com. Remember that you can always go back to using the apricots if you feel it would benefit you to use them.

One day when walking down the street,
On business bent, while thinking hard
About the "hundred cares" which seemed
Like thunder clouds about to break
In torrents, Self-pity said to me:
"You poor, poor thing, you have too much
To do. Your life is far too hard.
This heavy load will crush you soon."
A swift response of sympathy
Welled up within. The burning sun

Seemed more intense. The dust and noise
Of puffing motors flying past
With rasping blast of blowing horn
Incensed still more the whining nerves,
The fabled last back-breaking straw
To weary, troubled, fretting mind...
"Ah, yes, 'twill break and crush my life';
I cannot bear this constant strain
Of endless, aggravating cares;
They are too great for such as I."
So thus my heart condoled itself,
"Enjoying misery," when lo!
A **still small voice** *distinctly said,*
"'Twas sent to lift you—not to crush."
I saw at once my great mistake.
My place was not beneath the load
But on the top! God meant it not
That I should carry it. He sent
It here to carry me. Full well
He knew my incapacity
Before the plan was made. He saw
A child of His in need of grace
And power to serve; a puny twig
Requiring sun and rain to grow;
An undeveloped chrysalis;
A weak soul lacking faith in God.

He could not help but see all this
And more. And then with tender thought
He placed it where it had to grow
. . . To lie and cringe beneath
One's load means death, but life and power
Await all those who dare to rise above.
Our burdens are our wings; on them
We soar to higher realms of grace;
Without them we must roam for aye
On planes of undeveloped faith,
(For faith grows but by exercise
In circumstance impossible.)
Oh, paradox of Heaven. The load
We think will crush was sent to lift us
Up to God! Then, soul of mine
Climb up! For naught can e'er be crushed
Save what is underneath the weight.
How may we climb! By what ascent
Shall we surmount the carping cares
Of life! Within His word is found
The key which opens His secret stairs;
Alone with God, secluded there,
We mount our loads, and rest in Him.

—Miss Mary Butterfield

CHAPTER TWO

The Diagnosis We All Fear but Can Get Through Together

FINALLY, THE DAY FOR THE CORE BIOPSY ARRIVED. Thank God for Ahmad, who rubbed my feet throughout the entire process. I cannot suggest strongly enough that you have a relative or friend go with you, should you need to have this procedure done. To describe the core biopsy from someone who has had two of them: this is a very difficult and emotional procedure to go through. Actually, what hurt the most for me were the shots of local anesthesia. Hindsight says an initial shot of Valium certainly wouldn't have hurt.

The core biopsy needle was very long and nearly one-eighth inch in diameter. At the end of the needle was a round, quarter-inch-long piece that looked like a little weed-whacker. I almost fainted when I saw this instrument, knowing this was about to go into my breast. I covered my eyes with my hand. After the local anesthetic shots, which actually hurt more than the little weed-whacker needle, the doctor inserted the needle into the very core of my tumor. He continued to go into the core of my tumor about four or five times with the weed-whacker. All I felt was this "urrrrrr, urrrrrr, urrrrrr" each time he pulled out a little piece from the tumor, until he got all that he needed for the biopsy. When I asked to see the jar, I was amazed at how innocent and even pink those little buggers looked!

In my heart I prepared for the worst, but I acted as if everything would be fine. Ahmad and I then left, encouraged each other, and I went back to work so that I didn't have to think about everything I had just been through.

I got the results from the core biopsy the next morning. Again, I was at my parents' home when we called the biopsy doctor. The doctor confirmed my fears. He said, "I'm sorry to say that your lump has come back positive for breast cancer. It is an 'Infiltrating Ductal Carcinoma.' You'll need to call a breast surgeon immediately—here are a couple of references."

I was really not as much surprised as I was numb. I called Ahmad and told him, and he was not surprised either. Again, he said, "Honey, it's okay. We'll get through this together, no matter what. I love you for who you are—not for your breasts."

I think my breast cancer diagnosis was actually harder on my parents than on me because, in addition to their worry about me, all of this brought back memories for them of my mother's breast cancer forty years earlier. So my parents and I huddled and shed a few tears together. Actually, they shed most of the tears because I was still in shock.

Interestingly, in my mother's day, approximately forty-three years ago, there were only about 10,000 cases of breast cancer per year in America. Back in her day, if they found breast cancer on your breast they just lopped it off, and you woke up out of surgery without a breast. No questions asked. This is what my mother experienced, and there was no reconstruction in those days either. She was devastated—and my father was absolutely livid.

My father was a seasoned lawyer at that time and later became a Superior Court Judge. Immediately after the doctor informed my father that he had removed his wife's breast due to breast cancer, my father had the biopsy taken to UCLA to have it re-examined. Indeed, it was breast cancer and there was nothing they could do about it. So, my grandmother sent them on a two-week vacation to Hawaii. My mother is now a happy, healthy eighty-six-year-old survivor. In the last forty-three years they have traveled the world over, and they continue to have a wonderful life. My father views my mother's scar as a victory over a battle won.

Thankfully, within a couple of hours I was able to get an appointment with the breast surgeon.

"We have a little time to go out for coffee," I said to my mother, so off we went to Seattle's Best Coffee. I simply refused to be pessimistic, and believed that somehow everything would be okay. Out of concern, my best friend from childhood, Lisa, whom I hadn't seen in years, insisted on coming to the appointment with us. She met us there with her baby, which in fact added a little levity.

The breast surgeon was very sweet and comforting. She told me that I could have either a lumpectomy with radiation, or a mastectomy, and I'd probably still have to have radiation. "It's really up to you," she said.

"These days," she added, "we have found that lumpectomies with radiation, and possibly chemotherapy, have about the same result as mastectomies."

"Excuse me," I said, "did you say chemotherapy?"

"Yes. Well, I'm sorry to say that most breast cancer patients must have chemotherapy unless they are in Stage I, and even then sometimes they still have to have it."

"Well, if I get a mastectomy," I thought, "I won't have to have chemotherapy."

Upon asking her, she said, "That is not necessarily the case, depending on the size of the tumor and whether or not it has spread to the lymph nodes."

I knew that I had a lot ahead of me. I could be happy or be miserable. Either way, I was going to have to go through whatever was necessary to get through this, so I decided I was going to be strong.

Dissolving Into a Puddle

I went home to my boyfriend and I just lost it. We hugged each other and both of us cried. I could not believe this was happening to me, to us, and I felt like my whole world was coming apart at the seams.

He encouraged me, saying, "It's okay, sweetheart, we'll get through this together. You are not your breasts." We dealt with the diagnosis of breast cancer the only way we knew how; we cried and prayed a lot. This was the first time I had dissolved into a puddle. Unfortunately, it certainly wasn't going to be the last time either.

It is important to remember, dissolving into a puddle of tears at some point is expected, and, at many points, will probably occur throughout your journey. If you have a nervous breakdown or two, just remember you're not alone. You'll be okay, and it's quite normal under circumstances like this.

Going through breast cancer and chemotherapy is also a humbling time. In order for you to get through all of this with your sanity intact, you must reach out and ask for help. I guarantee someone will gently guide you.

Remember, no one ever died from crying, or even from sobbing. Just know that eventually the sun will come out and will dry up the puddle. As we all know, tears are cleansing and they will help you along your journey, whether you realize it or not. Tears will actually save your sanity rather than take it away, which so many of us fear. It is the people who refuse to cry that you have to worry about.

A little card written by Thomas McDermitt helped me many times. His introduction states, "You don't have to agree with all of this message all of the time. But, if it generally speaks to you, try to read all or parts of it every day, or have it read to you. Part of the help is in the doing, regardless of your attitude or emotions on that day. On some levels, the help is gradual."

Daily Survival Kit for Those with Serious Illness

BY THOMAS MCDERMITT

(a long-time cancer patient and skeptic)

1. Today I am going to try to live through this day only, and not dwell on or attempt to solve all my problems at once; just focus on the piece that is today. I can do something for several hours that would be difficult to even think about continuing for several months.

2. Just for today, I am willing to accept the possibility that there is a purpose to this suffering; that it can be a source of meaning and growth for me and others, though I may not always recognize the ways. And it seems possible that this suffering will not be in vain, because of what may be some kind of existence beyond.

3. Just for today, let me remind myself that I am basically a worthwhile person, worth loving, despite my faults and limits. I deserve the efforts of others to help me through my illness.

4. Just for today, I want to be aware that it is all right to want too much from others at times. Illness brings out and intensifies the small child in all of us. And if I feel hurt when those who care for me cannot be there, it may help to remember that they have needs, frailties, and limitations of their own. A lack of response does not mean that they are personally rejecting me.

5. Today I may feel the need to complain a great deal; I may have little tolerance; I may cry; I may scream. That does not mean that I am less courageous or strong. All are ways of expressing anger over this mess, of rightly mourning my losses. Endurance itself is courage.

6. It is my life that is at stake now. So maybe today I can allow myself to be a little less concerned about the reactions or impressions of others. Maybe I can allow myself to feel a little less guilty or bad about what I did not accomplish or give. Perhaps today I can be a little gentler toward myself.

7. Surviving this is all so difficult. At times it seems impossible—that I have had enough. Down the line I will know if and when I have had enough, when I cannot push the limits any further. I will have the right to choose to stop, without feeling that I am "giving up." But today I think I can deal with this illness. Sorrow runs very deep, but I think I can rise again.

8. Just for today, maybe I can give healing "the benefit of the doubt." The drugs are powerful; the natural healing capacity of my body is powerful. And who knows, perhaps there is healing power in my will to struggle, and in the collective love and will of others.

9. Just for today, perhaps I can take heart that we are all connected. And I may still have some things left to contribute to the family of man, some light to add to the light. Even now my endurance (however imperfect) is a gift, an inspiration for others in their struggles.

10. It seems reasonable that there is a season for everything, and a time for everything, and a time for every purpose. Pain, weakness and exhaustion may distort my senses and spirit. Today, however, I can at least find some hope in nature's way, if not in some master plan. The chances are fairly good, and it seems worthwhile to hope that I will have some cycle of wellness yet.

Belief in a Greater Power

Most of us start praying a lot more when we're in a situation of the unknown, or we at least begin seeking to find God or something of a higher power if we have never done so before. This is a time to find or renew your faith in whatever it is you choose to believe in. It is also a time to strengthen your faith. I am a Christian, so I read the Bible and other books that I find inspirational. My husband is a Muslim; I respect his beliefs highly and he respects mine. In fact sometimes we pray together, but mostly we pray on our own.

There is only one road to lead to God—humility.

—Nicholas Boileau

Study, Study, Study

We all know the saying, "knowledge is power." In order to feel you have some control over your disease it is important to study up on your particular breast cancer. In 2001, as soon as my father found out I had Stage 2B breast cancer, he became so worried that he ordered a 500-page publication for me entitled, *Treatments for Early Stage Breast Cancer* by The Health Resource Inc. It can be found online at, www.thehealthresource.com.

I immersed myself in every page. I cannot recommend it highly enough. I took out my yellow highlighter and devoured it over the first couple of months of my treatment, and I referred back to it many times when I was confused. It truly gave me all of the information I needed to understand my specific breast cancer and helped tremendously in my decision-making process regarding my treatment. The report answered literally any and all questions I had regarding my cancer, and it helped significantly in making decisions regarding my treatment. If you like to read and want to become more informed about your specific breast cancer, The Health Resource is definitely worth the investment.

The authors of the book, *Treatments for Early Stage Breast Cancer,* create information that is very specific to your particular type of breast cancer as well as other types of cancers upon request. It even had my name on the front cover which made me feel this book was made especially for me. It is a two-inch thick, 8 x 10 inch volume of research on the patient's specific breast cancer, and gives all of the various treatments for your cancer, testimonials, alternative medicines, etc.

Also, I highly suggest you learn how to read your pathology report. It will help you feel that you have more control over what is going on within you and around you, and will also help you make informed decisions regarding your treatment. One way to learn to read a pathology report is to ask your doctor to explain it to you. You can also learn by studying a breast cancer glossary of terms, but usually you will still need to talk to a professional to truly understand your pathology report. You can find a glossary of breast cancer terms at www.bca.ns.ca/glossary/.

CHAPTER THREE

Medical and Emotional Factors to Consider When Dealing with Breast Cancer

Meeting an Oncologist

MY MOTHER AND I IMMEDIATELY WENT TO MEET with an oncologist to determine my fate: whether or not I'd have to have chemo. The oncologist was known to be "one of the best," yet, neither my mother nor I could stand her. She appeared to be detached, telling me with her "cemented on" smile that I would have to have chemo with four rounds of treatment every three weeks, lose my hair, and be sick for at least four days after every treatment. Whether she was right or wrong, I knew I never wanted to see her again.

Meeting the Right Oncologist

Your first meeting with your selected oncologist is naturally kind of scary, as you don't know what they're going to say. I highly suggest that you bring someone with you because you will not remember everything the doctor says. I recommend that you have your spouse, boyfriend, or friend take notes for you. You can even ask the doctor if you can tape the consultation, if you'd like. This is a very emotional time, and because you will not remember everything the doctor says, make sure someone is there with you.

Since my insurance had just kicked in, Ahmad and I met with the woman who would become my oncologist. Her name is Dr. Kanchana Anand. She was just great for me. She was down to earth, very compassionate, and very patient. She told me that the chemo would probably knock out my periods since I was over forty. She let me cry as much as I needed to. She said that if I wanted to have a baby we'd have to get embryos frozen as soon as possible. She gave us the name of a fertility specialist to whom she often referred breast cancer patients. She said, as all the oncologists do, that I should wait two to five years before getting pregnant because the first two years are the highest risk for recurrence.

I wanted a fertility expert to guide us in the process of making embryos, and then have the embryos frozen until I was done with my treatment. However, since my breast cancer was estrogen-positive Ahmad did not want to risk my cancer coming back and so did not agree to the idea. Well, what was I going to do? I wasn't about to use a sperm donor. Although for some that is a wonderful idea, it just wasn't for me. I was in a committed relationship. The oncologist wanted me to start the chemo as soon as possible, so I just took it as a sign from God that maybe the door to having my own children was slowly being shut. I didn't have much time to think, let alone cry about it.

She actually spent forty-five minutes talking to us, answering all of our questions, and calming all our fears. The interesting thing was that she said the exact same thing as the first oncologist, but this time the words were much more palatable. She was definitely the right oncologist for me.

A Lumpectomy or a Mastectomy?

There was a scar on yonder mountain-side,
Gashed out where once the cruel storm had trod;
A barren, desolate chasm, reaching wide
Across the soft green sod.

But years crept by beneath the purple pines,
And veiled the scar with grass and moss once more
And left it fairer now with flowers and vines
Than it had been before.

There was a wound once in a gentle heart,
Whence all life's sweetness seemed to ebb and die;
And love's confiding changed to bitter smart,
While slow, sad years went by.

Yet as they passed, unseen an angel stole
And laid a balm of healing on the pain,
Till love grew purer in the heart made whole,
And peace came back again.

— Unknown

"Okay, well, let's see. I'm now forty-one, never been married, currently have a boyfriend who I've been with for a year. Um, should I have a mastectomy? Are you kidding? No way! Then for sure no one would love me." Both Ahmad and my father wanted me to get a mastectomy. I asked them, "How would you like it if someone cut off one of your testicles, and gave you a fake one?" Well, that was much more difficult for them to respond to. So I had a lumpectomy, chemo and radiation.

I later learned that a mastectomy no longer has to make a woman look or feel disfigured. In fact, many breast cancer patients feel that they now have better looking breasts than they had before! Due to state laws requiring the option of reconstructive surgery with a mastectomy, a woman can have beautifully reconstructed breasts after a mastectomy. In 2004, when my breast cancer returned I found out that the radiated breast is much more difficult for reconstructive plastic surgeons to work with. Still, if you choose to have a mastectomy either before or after having radiation, there are many options for your reconstruction.

I will not doubt, though all my ships at sea
Come drifting home with broken masts and sails;
I will believe the Hand which never fails,
From seeming evil worketh good for me.
And though I weep because those sails are tattered,
Still will I cry, while my best hopes lie shattered:
'I trust in Thee.'

I will not doubt, though all my prayers return
Unanswered from the still, white realm above;
I will believe it is an all-wise love
Which has refused these things for which I yearn;
And though at times I cannot keep from grieving,
Yet the pure ardor of my fixed believing
Undimmed shall burn.

I will not doubt, though sorrow fall like rain,
And troubles swarm like bees about a hive.
I will believe the heights for which I strive
Are only reached by anguish and by pain;

And though I groan and write beneath my crosses,
I yet shall see through my severest losses
The greater gain.

—Unknown

If you have had a radiated breast, however, just know that most doctors are not willing to put implants into a radiated breast because the radiated tissue inside the breast becomes tougher, making the entire breast more difficult to expand. If you do have a radiated breast, you may want to choose a different reconstructive option than implants, and that will be discussed later. Luckily, I did find a doctor in Beverly Hills, Dr. Linda Li, who was willing to take the chance and to put the expanders in my radiated breast after my double mastectomy so that I could have implants.

It would be of benefit for you to know that a radiated breast takes three to four times longer to expand than a non-radiated breast. If you have had radiation and want implants, you will have to be very patient with the process. One very good secret for exapanding radiated skin is to twice a day for a couple of minutes massage the outer perimeter of the breast with Vitamin E. Still, depending on the breast size you want, it can take up to a year or even a little more for the radiated breast to get to that size, if it can even reach it! You must realize that the radiated breast may not be able to stretch beyond a size B bra. It will also be a little harder to the touch than the non-radiated breast, but it sure can look beautiful, just like the other one.

So if you want implants despite radiation, you will have to find a good reconstructive plastic surgeon that will be willing to do that for you. Don't be fooled that just because your radiated breast is still supple, it will expand normally. My radiated breast is still a little smaller than my non-radiated breast, but my doctor and I are hoping that after another year or more the tissue of the radiated breast will thicken and be strong enough to withstand a larger implant. If or until that time comes, I am happy just wearing Wonderbras which make both breasts look the same size. I could have my non-radiated breast made smaller, but I love it just the way it is.

If you have radiation after you have your implant(s), the radiation may affect the cosmetic look of the breast. It will also increase the possibility of "capsular contraction," which is scar tissue that can form around a breast implant and make it feel hard and sometimes painful as well. The possible need for removal of the implant may even arise. So these are things you definitely need to consider and discuss with your doctor when deciding what kind of breast surgery and treatment you will have.

If you have, or will have a radiated breast, many breast surgeons will recommend you have what is known as the DIEP flap reconstruction where they use the skin and fat on your abdomen to fill the breast. A positive aspect of this procedure is that they spare the abdominal muscles. A second option your breast surgeon may recommend is the TRAM flap or "tummy tuck" breast reconstruction if you have enough fat on your stomach to be transferred to your breasts. They transfer skin, fat, and a portion of the abdominal muscle to the breast. There are also several other reconstructive techniques. All of these reconstructive techniques need to be thoroughly discussed with your doctor in order for you to understand the pros and cons, as well as which surgery would be appropriate for you.

Fertility Issues

The question of whether or not to have a baby is actually a question no one can decide except you yourself. Although Ahmad had been open to having another child (he has two teenage girls from a previous marriage), he said that it was more important to him that I follow the doctor's instructions and stay alive than that we have a child of our own together. Although I loved his girls, I still thought that having my own baby was essential to my happiness. I now have come to believe that acceptance is the key to happiness.

Your oncologist will make strong recommendations, but the decision as to whether or not to have a baby is ultimately up to you. Again, oncologists want you to wait two to five years after your treatment is complete before trying to have a baby because the first two years have the highest risk of recurrence. So if you definitely want to have a baby, consider having embryos frozen before your chemo. You won't have much time to contemplate this decision, however, as they usually want to start chemo within a month after your lumpectomy or mastectomy. If you are in your twenties or early thirties chances are that your periods will return after your treatment and you will still be fertile.

There is good news if you are already pregnant. According to *Cure Magazine,* the discovery was recently made that: "Although it was initially believed that pregnant breast cancer patients did not fare as well as non-pregnant patients, it is now believed that there is no difference in survival when comparing pregnant with non-pregnant patients with the same stage of breast cancer" (*Cure Magazine*, Winter 2005 p.59).

Will My Sex Life Change? Retaining Your Sexual Dignity

No matter which treatment you need to go through, you cannot get through breast cancer without questioning how the treatments will affect your sex life and your sense of sexuality. Regardless of your age, when you get breast cancer and begin to go through the treatments, your sexual drive will likely decline and your sexual confidence may therefore be under siege. Depending on your age and the type of treatment that you will need to go through, there are different stages of what one might call "sexual crisis." Also, don't be surprised if some sexual issues arise throughout various treatments.

Remember that no matter whether you have insurance or financial means or not, it has become a law in most states that reconstruction must be offered. If you cannot find a hospital in your state that provides free reconstruction and you cannot afford it, you can use the Corporate Angel Network mentioned in the Free Assistance Programs chapter to get to the treatment center that will best meet your needs.

When a woman has chemo and she's pre-menopausal, she may naturally wonder whether or not she will be able to have children. The younger she is, usually the less sex drive she will lose during treatment. Then, whether she is pre-menopausal or post-menopausal, if she ends up having to have a single or a bilateral mastectomy, she may likely wonder whether or not she will be able to attract or keep a man even if she has reconstruction.

All of this is perfectly natural. Remember that *you* are not your breasts, your ovaries, or your fertility. Depending on whether your cancer is estrogen-positive or estrogen-negative, that will certainly be a factor as to whether or not your doctor will allow you any kind of natural hormone replacement therapy. If you are estrogen-positive, your doctor will be unlikely to recommend any kind of hormone replacement therapy even if it is the non-synthetic Bioidentical Hormone Replacement therapy that Suzanne Sommers promotes, because that also stimulates estrogen production. You may want to try a lubricant called "Astroglide," or for a longer lasting lubricant you can try "Replens". Both are helpful for those who may experience painful sex due to lack of lubrication.

If you are estrogen-negative, Bioidentical Hormone Replacement therapy may be an option for you. You can discuss these natural remedies with your doctors and see what they recommend. Whichever you choose, breast cancer treatment does affect sexual desire, and it is best if we come to a place of acceptance of that. Many times this lack of sex drive is temporary and will return the closer you get to your treatments being completed, including any adjuvant treatment pills you may be recommended to take.

If you want to maintain your sex drive as much as is physically possible during treatment, you might consider consulting with a certified nutritionist to keep yourself happy and retain your sexual desire. Remember that having sex and retaining your sexual dignity are not one and the same. You must accept whatever place of sexual desire you are at during any given time. Don't let anyone push you by trying to make you feel guilty for not wanting to have sex at their convenience. If you do that you will surely lose your sexual dignity.

For many of us, our sex life is important to our happiness. Each of us needs to pursue what is right for ourselves. At the same time, as we all know, true love is not based on sex. Believe it or not, there are many happy marriages out there that are mostly celibate due to various reasons and various choices.

If you are still on the dating scene, I would recommend that you don't start dating again until after your major treatments are done. Dating will probably be the last thing on your mind during this time anyway. When you do start dating again, I would recommend that you do not disclose your breast cancer status until at least two to six weeks into the relationship. I have talked to several men about this, and they said that they would rather wait to hear that information so that they can make an informed decision about starting a serious relationship.

Truly, the only way to get through all of this is to talk to your breast cancer "sisters" about it. All the help you need is out there.

Free Assistance Programs

As a breast cancer patient, if you want to have your treatment performed in a state other than your own, you and your family can fly for free with Corporate Angel Network. "CAN" is a national public charity that works directly with cancer patients and their families, assisting them in coordinating flight plans on corporate jets to recognized treatment centers around the country.

Corporate Angel Network (CAN) is funded by many of the nation's top 500 companies including 56 of the top 100 *Fortune 500* companies. They happen to have aircraft that are only half full, and they consider this an opportunity to give a cancer patient a lift both in body and spirit. You can find them at Info@CorpAngelNetwork.org or www.CorpAngelNetwork.org. You can also give them a call in the U.S. at (914) 328-1313 or toll free at (866) 328-1313. They promise to do all the work for you so that you and your family can travel for free to the treatment center that you and your doctor believe would be best for you.

Also, if you are forty or older and do not have medical insurance, you may be able to get full or partial Medi-Cal through a program called "Every Woman Counts." Every Woman Counts provides free breast exams and mammograms for low-income, uninsured or underinsured breast cancer patients. You can find them at www.vchca.org/ph/ed/cdp-ewc/index.htm. If you do not qualify, the regional cancer detection partnership in your area may know of other low-income screening programs.

Animal Therapy—Dad's Gift

Sometimes when we have no clue as to what to do, our parents know just what we need. My dad knew I needed a puppy and was determined to buy me one. He asked me what kind I wanted. I wanted a Maltese, so we looked in the newspaper and drove over an hour to see the cutest puppies I had ever seen. I chose the one I wanted, and since both the puppy and I are Italian, I named him "Piccolo," which in Italian means the tiniest musical flute.

I cannot emphasize enough the importance of the role that this puppy has played in my life. He was about three months old and he needed nurturing just as much as I did. We nurtured each other. There is nothing like a puppy to comfort you when you are going through chemo. He was not ready to be walked, and I was not ready to walk him, so Ahmad and I taught him to "tee-tee" on the newspaper, which worked great for all of us.

When I was finished with my chemo and radiation, I began to walk Piccolo two or three times a day. I needed the walks just as much as he did. In fact, honestly, I would not have gone out of the house or done any exercise if it were not for Piccolo.

When you have a dog you must usually walk him twice a day. Your love for him or her can be just the right motivation you need to get out and get some fresh air as well as a little exercise. Remember to get a puppy, or any other type of animal, that is known to be a friendly breed, so that you don't scare all your friends and family away. Also, make sure that in your heart you are willing to commit to taking care of your animal for its entire life. Believe me, simply having an animal does wonders for your inspiration, motivation, and sense of purpose when you are going through breast cancer.

POWER OF SELF
I Did It for a Very Good Friend of Mine, Which Happened to be Me

I absolutely could not believe this was happening to me. So, I decided in my heart that I was going to go through all of this for a very good friend of mine. This good friend happened to be me. I resolved to get my "friend" the best treatment, and I was going to nurture her like she so much deserved because she was my good friend.

So, a week later after my diagnosis on October 23, 2001, which is also Breast Cancer Month, I had my lumpectomy—for her. I am very thankful for her that it did not spread to the lymph nodes. The breast surgeon told me that it was a Stage 2B out of four stages. I was thankful for my friend that it was in the latest of the early stages. The doctor said the size of the tumor was

2.5 centimeters, or one inch for those of us who, like me, are not very good at math.

I began to wonder if the way the doctor who used the "weed-whacker" for initial biopsy had caused my breast to become inflamed. But no such luck, said the oncologist. Either way, I was still thankful for my good friend that, although the tumor was the most aggressive kind that exists, it had not spread to the lymph nodes!

Giving Service to Others

When all else fails and you are so depressed that you don't know what to do with yourself, I suggest you get out and help someone else. If you do that, you will quickly find how much one act can work miracles in your own life! When I became really depressed I would walk over to my frail eight-four-year-old aunt's apartment. Her health was declining fairly rapidly. All she needed was someone to talk with her, maybe make her a couple of meals, and give her a bath if the daycare help didn't arrive. It never failed that I felt much better after having helped her even just a little bit.

Your journey through breast cancer is a time to be with family and friends. You will find out how much people care about you. I highly recommend finding a breast cancer group through your local hospital that you can try to attend weekly. Again, I reiterate the importance of finding a website for women who are going through, or have already been through breast cancer. Believe me, there are many women with breast cancer that make terrific use of the websites that are out there. Those women can help you like no one else can, because there is nothing like chatting with someone who has gone through—or is going through—the same diagnosis and treatment as you are. It really becomes like a "sisterhood."

Other times, when I was feeling sorry for myself, I would call someone from my breast cancer group who I knew was having a more difficult time than I was. We would just chat each other out of our self pity. We all have friends, relatives, or neighbors who would love to come over and bring something we want from the grocery store or maybe just help get our laundry done. Allow people the chance to be blessed by helping you!

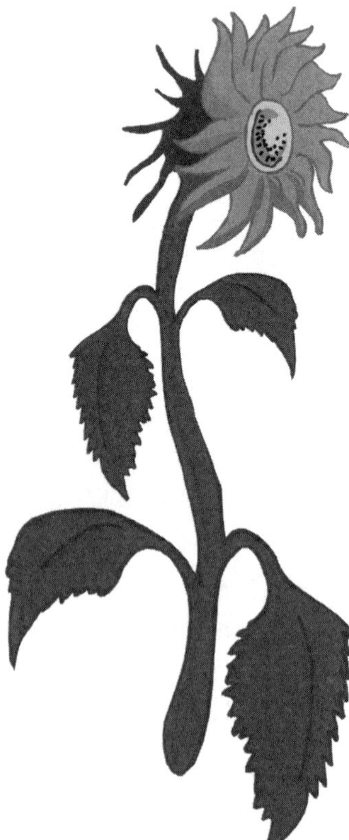

CHAPTER FOUR

Preparing for Chemo with All the Necessary Accessories

I'm Losing My Hair!

FORTUNATELY, NOT ALL CHEMOTHERAPY CAUSES HAIR LOSS. However, many, if not most do. You will want to ask your oncologist if your chemo will cause hair loss. If you have the type of chemo that causes hair loss, there are many beautiful wigs and hats out there for you to use. The chemo I had was Adriomycin with Cytoxin or "AC," the name by which it is more commonly known. My mother and I went to a little boutique at UCLA for cancer patients called "Reflections." The wig lady said, "Oh, if you are going to have 'AC' then you will definitely lose your hair, so let me help you find a nice wig." She was very sweet and very patient. She helped me try on all the wigs I wanted until I found the perfect one for me. The one I chose looked a lot like the hair I already had, but the cut was just a little more stylish. Then I bought a hat to go with it. My mother and I were having so much fun that the wig lady said jokingly, "You guys are just having too much fun." We then went out to lunch and made a day of it.

In preparing for chemotherapy, you definitely will first of all need a snuggly sleeper hat. The reason for this is that your head will get cold at night, which can cause your whole body to feel cold. Also, it will make you feel more comfortable and secure in your cozy bed. I ordered my very cute snuggly pink sleeper hat from chemosavvy.com. They have lots of very nice hats and wigs as well.

If you, like me, decide to go out on the town to find a wig, you will want to go with a family member or a friend. It's not much fun going alone. Most hospitals can refer you to very nice, affordable places to buy wigs. Also, insurance companies are now required to pay for a wig if you have cancer. In wig shops that specifically cater to cancer patients, you will find the people very friendly and helpful. Most of us end up buying a wig that looks like our own hair, but if you're blonde or brunette and want to be a redhead—go for it! Then go out to lunch with your family member or friend and make a day of it.

It is always good to cut your hair very short a couple of weeks before you know it will fall out. This lessens the trauma of hair loss to some degree. When you know it is time to shave your head, make an evening out of it. Have a loved one cut your hair while you are sipping on a glass of wine. If you feel comfortable, invite a couple of very close friends or relatives. Their support and unconditional acceptance does wonders when you have to shave your head.

Know that your hair, like mine, will grow back dancing! Most women who have temporary hair loss through chemo find that their hair returns with more volume and curls as well! The first couple of months after your chemo, you will get the "fuzzies" and begin to wonder if your hair will ever be normal again. The fuzzies are very normal. Within a couple of months after the fuzzies your hair will begin to thicken. For about the first half to one-half inch, it will look like it is going to be strong and straight. Then most women get "the curlies." It will not always necessarily be curly, however. After your hair continues to grow for a couple of years, it will look like a three or four-year-old girl's hair; the ends of the hair will become long and full of curls. Mine came out the same color, maybe even a little darker than it was before. And if you don't like the color, there's always the tint bottle to change your hair to whatever color you desire.

Obviously the longer you let your hair grow the less curls you'll have because of the weight of the hair. Since my chemo five years ago I have never cut my hair, so it is quite long and still a little curly at the ends. Some of us just don't want to cut our hair ever again after chemo, although one day I probably will.

Remember Your Eyebrows!

I happened to get my eyebrows tattooed six months before I knew I had cancer, and I was so happy I did that. It makes such a difference in your looks to have nice eyebrows. I suggest that you get them done *before* your chemotherapy so the cosmetologist can enhance your eyebrows just as they are and to avoid getting some type of infection. You will be happy you did. The tattoos will last anywhere from two to five years. One good thing to remember is that if they offer you a lighter or a darker color, always choose the lighter one. Even if you have dark brunette hair like I do, very dark eyebrows just don't look right when they have no hair on them. I chose a caramel color which worked perfectly for me. Remember, you can always darken your eyebrows with liner, but you can't lighten them.

Free Cosmetic Assistance Programs Available

There are wonderful free make-up and skin care gift boxes given when you go to a "Look Good…Feel Better" workshop supported by the American Cancer Society. "The Look Good…Feel Better" workshops are provided in many States. Times and locations for these workshops can be found by going to lookgoodfeelbetter.org. These free workshops are the result of many top department stores donating excellent make-up. Cosmetologists at the meeting will show you how to use the various products. You will meet others going through the same thing. Another part of this workshop that many find really fun is the gift boxes because each one is different. The cosmetologists who attend these workshops will try to match a facial foundation specifically for your skin type. They usually also provide a good sun block for underneath your make-up, because when you are in chemo your skin is more sensitive to the sun.

You will probably even make a friend or two during the workshop, as each person is encouraged to tell a little bit about themselves and their type of cancer.

What is the Chemo Room Like?

Most places that administer chemotherapy treatments have a room with comfortable lounge chairs and blankets. Most often chemotherapy is administered in a room with many other cancer patients also having chemo. The people in the chemo room are usually either reading a book, sleeping, listening to their Ipod, or they are quietly chatting with a loved one. When women go through chemo they can become very vulnerable and even childlike, because chemo treatments can be such an emotional experience. For many men and women, the loss of hair can be even worse than the nausea that accompanies chemo. You should always bring a family member or friend with you, not only to keep you company, but because you will not be allowed to drive home alone due to the necessary sedatives that are added to the chemo. According to my oncologist, the sedatives such as Ativan are "absolutely necessary" due to the stimulant ingredients in the chemo. She said that if I did not have a sedative in the I.V., I would be jumping to the ceiling. I found that to be very true, because when I went home and the sedative wore off, I began shaking and felt like I wanted to jump out of my skin. Fortunately, she had prescribed Ativan for me and that made me feel calm and normal again.

I am not an actress, but I do get a bit dramatic at times. My twin sister, Sharon, brought me to my second chemo treatment. She was so sweet. She wore all of her hair in a scarf to make *me* feel better. However, since I had just recently lost my hair and was experiencing many other fears, I began crying hysterically, asking for my doctor and screaming, "They're torturing me." A very nice older man said, "You're a fighter—you just fight!" He was so sweet he was like an angel to me. But I was beyond fighting. My poor twin sister tried her best to comfort me with her sweet words. If she couldn't comfort me no one could.

Following that outburst, I was kindly escorted to a private room where they finished giving me my chemo, because they did not want me upsetting the other patients. They also sent my oncologist, Dr. Kanchana Anand, who was able to comfort me and calm me down. After that experience, I was provided that private room each time I was administered chemotherapy. Because of the emotional and physical trauma of cancer and chemo, that type of reaction can be normal. You just don't read about it in the newspaper.

During my fourth and last chemo session I had my mother come and bring our childhood family album, plus I had her read me a Dr. Seuss book. That may seem extreme to some people, but it's sometimes how we get through things. It was how I wanted to end my chemotherapy, because I wanted to remember all the fun times in my childhood, and because I felt like I was like a child starting a new life.

CHAPTER FIVE

From Chemo to Radiation

AFTER YOUR LAST CHEMO TREATMENT you will more than likely be exhausted both physically and emotionally. You may even wonder how you are going to possibly have the energy to be driven or even shuttled daily to your radiation treatment. Because of this, check with your insurance company to see what accommodations they may have for you if you need to have radiation treatment. Unfortunately, most insurance companies do not usually voluntarily offer this information.

Luckily, a family member nudged us to call our HMO and find out what accommodations they might have for people needing radiation treatment. We were very lucky to have discovered that my HMO owned an apartment building specifically for those going through radiation who, for one reason or another, needed to live closer to the radiation treatment hospital. The apartments were free for the duration of radiation treatment, which was six and one-half weeks for us. That was truly a godsend.

So, for the duration of my radiation, we lived a block away from the radiation treatment hospital. I felt extremely blessed to have been able to obtain a free apartment a block away from the hospital. I considered it my "job" to walk to my radiation for my 7:47 a.m. appointment (they had very odd appointment hours because there were so many people to treat). Then I just rested for most of the day. That was the extent of my energy level. Three months later I felt well enough to go back to work, which I did.

What is Radiation Like?

Simply preparing you to receive radiation treatments is a very meticulous process. You will have a couple of appointments, one of which may take up to an hour or more, while they use large machines to measure, to the exact millimeter, where to radiate your breast. Then they "tattoo" several very tiny dots on your breast in order to make it easier for them to guarantee they are radiating the right place. I had radiation five days a week for six and one-half weeks. The nurses and technicians there were really nice, very patient and very understanding. The other patients in the waiting room were also most friendly and chatty because we all knew we were there for the same reason. I even looked forward to seeing some of them during the mornings of my radiation.

The radiation itself takes only a few minutes each day to complete. The technicians place a big round machine a couple of feet or so from your breast, and then you'll hear a little buzzer go on for a short amount of time. Because the radiation machine is so large it can feel quite intimidating. Those three minutes seemed like an eternity because I was distinctly reminded that I had breast cancer, which I was trying to forget. I would close my eyes and think of being on a beautiful beach. When I became more used to the process I would stare at a nice picture on the wall and silently sing a little song to myself to keep myself occupied. Ipods are also great to bring to listen to soothing music.

The Return and the Slaying of the Dragon

Around September 2004, I received a card in the mail that Dr. Armando Giuliano was giving a lecture on breast cancer in Santa Monica, California. I thought my breast cancer was over, so I hemmed and hawed about going. Then, on the day of the lecture my mother encouraged me to go and for some reason I felt I should. I went to the lecture and won the raffle, which was a free bone density test. This was sweet, but I was pretty sure I would never need that type of test.

Then the following month, I went to get my annual breast exam. The head nurse who performed the breast exam felt a lump, became angry, and in her Asian accent she reprimanded me and said, "Don you eva do bress exam?"

I said, "Yes, but this lump felt like the scar tissue from the lumpectomy."

She immediately sent me for a mammogram. Both Ahmad and my mother met me there. Interestingly, nothing came up on the mammogram. It is a known fact that if a woman is over forty, for whatever reason, her lump will often fail to show up on a mammogram. Therefore, if you feel a lump and you are over forty, you should always insist on an ultrasound.

Because of my previous history of breast cancer, and because we could clearly feel a lump, the doctor immediately ordered the technician to perform an ultrasound. There, just five centimeters from the lumpectomy scar, was another "suspicious finding—biopsy should be considered."

"Oh dear God, here we go again," I said to myself. I knew if it was positive for breast cancer I was in for a mastectomy this time.

Ahmad and I were able to make an appointment a week later with the same doctor we previously had at the Women's Breast Center in Santa Monica. And there we were to meet once again with the little weed-whacker for another core biopsy. Not so surprisingly, the pathology report came back positive for breast cancer. I knew I hadn't been diligent with taking my Tamoxifin. Again, I had only taken it for about eight months because I wanted to get pregnant. Still it is always a shock when breast cancer returns. All of the fears of what might lay ahead came flooding into my brain. Luckily, the cancer still had not spread so I did not have to have chemo again.

Since my previous breast surgeon had moved out of state, we had to interview and find a new breast surgeon. We were blessed to be recommended to Dr. Bret Taback, who at that time worked with Dr. Giuliano in Santa Monica, California. Dr. Taback was also conducting breast cancer research at Good Samaritan Hospital in Los Angeles. He recommended a single mastectomy and said he could spare my other breast for the sake of being able to feel it during intimacy, and he said the plastic surgeon could match the breasts.

I told him I wanted a double mastectomy with expanders with subsequent implants because I didn't want to risk the cancer sneaking into the other breast, and I wanted to make sure my breasts matched. He recommended plastic reconstructive surgeon, Dr. Linda Li.

Like most reconstructive surgeons Dr. Li was hesitant to put an implant in a radiated breast because it is so much harder to expand, and it is a bit harder to the touch. However, my breast was supple enough that, thankfully, she gave it a chance. Although I was given the choice of silicone implants, after reviewing the pros and cons Ahmad and I chose the saline implants. I must say the implants look incredibly beautiful and Ahmad thinks so too!

Dr. Li was present at the double mastectomy surgery in December 2004. She put the expanders in after Dr. Taback performed the surgery. After the surgery, Dr. Taback told me the tumor had not spread to the lymph nodes and said he believed I had a 95 percent chance of a cure prognosis. The dragon was slain, and both he and I knew it!

I was so grateful to have such a good prognosis and to have the surgery over with. My breasts were still flat as a board, or more like a pancake, because the expanders had been placed, but not inflated. I knew that Dr. Li would fill the expanders with saline approximately every three weeks until I was the size I wanted to be. Within four months, the non-radiated breast expanded to the size I wanted, but the radiated breast took a little over a year.

Ahmad and I decided to exchange the expanders for implants four months after the double mastectomy. I used what is called a "poof" in my bra until the radiated breast was nearly the same size as the non-radiated breast. Filling implants is kind of like a pregnancy where the skin expands slowly with time. Also, until the permanent implant is inserted, there is a little valve in the saline implant where the doctor can put more saline in but no saline will come out.

About a year after my double mastectomy, everything was more beautiful than I had imagined it to be, which always reminded me of the following poem. (I have substituted the original "he" with "she".)

It Couldn't Be Done

Somebody said that it couldn't be done,
But she with a chuckle replied
That "maybe it couldn't," but she would be one
Who wouldn't say so till she'd tried.
So she buckled right in with the trace of a grin
On her face. If she worried she hid it.
She started to sing as she tackled the thing
That couldn't be done, and she did it.

Somebody scoffed: "Oh, you'll never do that
At least no one ever has done it."
But she took off her coat and she took off her hat,
And the first thing we knew she'd begun it.
With a lift of her chin and a bit of a grin,
Without any doubting or quiddit,
She started to sing as she tackled the thing
That couldn't be done, and she did it.

There are thousands to tell you it cannot be done,
There are thousands to prophesy failure;
There are thousands to point out to you, one by one,
The dangers that wait to assail you.
But just buckle in with a bit of a grin,

Just take off your coat and go to it;
Just start to sing as you tackle the thing
That "cannot be done," and you'll do it.
—EDGAR GUEST

Handling the Stress of Paying the Bills

Don't worry; you are not alone with feeling stressed simply when a bill arrives. Whether you have the money to pay your bills or not, just writing out checks while going through breast cancer treatment can be like trying to write with your left hand if you are right-handed and vice versa. Questions like, "Why is the world still demanding of me?" or, "Don't they know that I have cancer and am having a very rough time?" arise. Well, unfortunately "they" don't, and the bills from wherever will continue to come in.

If you have a spouse or a friend who is willing to write out the checks for you, this can relieve a lot of stress. If you are unable to pay your bills, simply call the company and let them know the situation you are currently dealing with. The people on the other line are human too and they will usually do what they can to try to reduce your monthly payments. If you can afford an accountant to do your bills, by all means do this. I cannot emphasize enough the relief this kind of help can give you.

Implants: Silicone Now a Solid "Maybe"

According to the *Los Angeles Times* November 18, 2006 issue, "the FDA rescinded a fourteen-year ban on silicone gel for cosmetic use... Several prominent female lawmakers expressed doubts on the decision. This appears to be yet another example of the FDA dismissing scientific evidence in order to appease corporate interests, said DeLauro, who is in line to chair the panel that controls the FDA's purse strings...Newer implants have been redesigned. However, the FDA states that implants are subject to breakdown and that women need to be tested regularly after surgery."

According to Diana M. Zuckerman, president of the National Research Center for Women & Families, an advocacy group that opposed the decision: "The message to women is let the buyer beware...Please understand that the FDA has not concluded that breast implants are safe, they have only concluded that they are 'reasonably safe,' and that's not much assurance."

According to the *Los Angeles Times* November 17, 2006 issue, the American Society of Plastic Surgeons' public education representative, Dr. Walter Erhardt, said that the (FDA) agency's decision "does create a whole host of questions" for women considering silicone breast augmentation and for the doctors who perform those procedures...Patients intent on getting silicone implants "really look on the bright side of the controversy," he said. "Although many prospective patients will inquire, my recommendation to them may not be to have surgery (with silicone breast implants) at this time," he added.

Silicone implants use to be the standard until the FDA imposed a moratorium on them in 1992, meaning that silicone implants would no longer be available for the general public. Since 1992, due to safety concerns, a moratorium remained on women receiving silicone implants unless the women wanting them could meet certain requirements. The reason for this strict requirement was because of an ongoing controversy concerning silicone breast implants and their connection to women contracting Connective Tissue Disorders (CTD) as well as other disorders. The symptoms of CTD usually include capsular contraction, rupture of the implant(s) and breast pain. However, silicone gel implants are approved for women who have had a mastectomy and agree to participate in a five to ten year follow-up study.

Autoimmune system complications can be another one of the major problems of silicone implants. Autoimmune system complications happen when a slow leakage ("bleeding") of the silicone gel seeps from the implants through the semi-permeable membrane envelope and also into and through the capsule that surrounds the implants. The gel eventually breaks down and causes the cells to travel all over the body. This causes immune system dysregulation ruptures, deflations, capsular contracture, infection, and pain. Many women will have secondary problems such as severe contracture, rupture, and eventual implant removal.

Implants do not last forever. Risks do accumulate over time, and many women should expect to have more than one implant. However if the silicone implants do not cause a problem, they do not need to be removed.

The Food and Drug Administration still does not approve silicone breast implants for cosmetic surgery, because they believe there is not enough evidence to support long-term safety and all of the design problems that have caused many implants to break within five years. Despite the gel silicone implants, leakage can still occur in the body causing various problems. Many women believe their silicone implants have caused severe problems to their lungs due to implant leakage.

Others are concerned about Chronic Fatigue Syndrome which may occur as a result of silicone implant leakage. In contrast, if a saline implant ruptures, say, due to a car accident, the rupture is obvious because the implant(s) will quickly deflate and only harmless salt water will disperse into your system. However, ruptures of silicone implants are not usually noticeable by feel or by the naked eye. Silicone can seep from ruptured implants and leak into the lymph glands, and it can also bleed from intact implants. Then there also is the chance of "silicone anxiety" after women study up on their implants.

Panel members have therefore been concerned about the reliability of silicone implants. Some studies have found that the probability of rupture by the tenth year ranged from 5 percent to 29 percent for cosmetic surgery patients and from 39 percent to 95 percent for cancer patients having breast reconstruction. Now that's a huge difference in statistics! Unfortunately most of the panel members do not know why the silicone implants fail when they do.

Interestingly, women interested in choosing silicone implants must sign a 20-page document full of disclaimers informing them of the side effects that they may experience if choosing silicone implants. Thus, the manufacturer protects themselves so that they will not be held responsible for any problems that may happen as a result of using silicone gel implants. The major manufacturers of silicone gel implants are: Mentor, Silimed and Dow Corning. If you come across a website that has these names in it, I suggest you search another website as well, because the major manufacturers' reports may be biased for obvious reasons, as well as reasons including investments in stock.

My husband and I decided that I would get saline implants so we would not have to worry about any of the above-mentioned problems. Saline implants don't have "silent ruptures." If the saline implant were to leak due to a car accident or a harsh blow to the breast, saline is just salt water and will not affect your body in any way. Also, it would be obvious if you had a saline leakage, because your breast would completely deflate. Then you would just have a new one put in to replace it. You might be embarrassed in front of the paramedics, but other than that you would not have to worry about all the possible ingredients that silicone implants have that could affect your body.

Unlike what the manufacturers of silicone will tell you, saline implants are absolutely beautiful. I can't tell you how happy I am that I made that decision. It's just one less thing to worry about. However, if you choose silicone implants, I hope by the time you do they are much more reliable and less risky. God knows we have enough to worry about without having to worry that the implants we have chosen are dangerous to our health.

The Task of Driving

For many of us who are going through breast cancer treatment, driving can become very uncomfortable. This is not only because of the medications being taken, but also because of the mental and emotional stress a patient is experiencing while undergoing the disease of cancer and cancer treatments. I felt very shaky driving throughout my treatment and even a couple of months beyond. I got two speeding tickets in one month. I rarely ever get a ticket, let alone one for speeding. My driving record was as clean as a whistle. I tried to cry my way out of the second one by letting the officer know I was going through breast cancer and that I was wearing a wig, but it didn't work. Maybe I should have taken my wig off when he came back to give me the ticket. Oh well.

Although I am very sociable, I was not in the mood to attend traffic school at that time. So I completed traffic school through a videotape I rented. I answered the questions online to get myself off of one of the tickets. Then, rather than driving, I began walking to places I needed to go, or I asked a family member to drive me. I waited a couple of months to start driving again. I waited until I felt sane enough so as not to be a hazard to myself or others.

Oh My Aching Joints and Bones!

Estrogen is the protective hormone that blocks bone loss. When we start losing estrogen, we start losing bone density. If you are taking Tamoxifin, Arimidex or Femara, sooner or later you will experience joint and sometimes bone aches starting most often in the mornings. The medications mentioned above are attempting to rid your body of estrogen which fuels breast cancer. Thus, we start having joint pain and sometimes bone pain. Joint and bone pain are very irritating and uncomfortable as well as emotionally troubling when we are fairly young or feel we are fairly young.

Regardless of your age, I cannot emphasize enough if you have been through chemo and are on adjuvant treatment that you drink three glasses of milk and take 1500 mg of calcium with 400 mg of Vitamin D daily. That is because the chemo begins to strip you of your estrogen, which will eventually cause bone loss. So even if you're young and think you're invincible, you need to be smart to avoid osteoporosis at all costs. Remember to drink your milk and take your calcium.

At the beginning of 2005 I started taking Arimidex, which is for estrogen-positive post-menopausal women. I was not completely post-menopausal yet, but very near it because of the chemo. The oncologist assured me that I would begin to enter menopause immediately after I began taking the prescribed medications. Not only was I given Arimidex, I was also prescribed monthly painful shots in my tummy, called Zoladex, just to ensure that my periods would stop. If you must have this shot, make sure you get a local shot of anesthesia beforehand. Trust me, you'll be happy you did.

Because Arimidex causes bone loss, I was very thankful for the free bone density test I won at the conference raffle in September 2004, a time when I still did not even know that my breast cancer had recurred. To my surprise when I received the bone density test in 2005, I was at the very beginning stages of Osteopenia, a term I didn't even know existed. Basically, bone density goes like this: 1) Normal, 2) Osteopenia, and then 3) Osteoporosis. I started taking restorative bone enhancer, called Fosamax. However, due to allegations that Fosamax causes necrosis of the jaw bone, I stopped it. Sometimes just drinking milk and taking calcum is the best and safest way to go. I am now cancer-free at this point, and the Osteopenia is reversing itself, so whatever I am asked to do, I will, and I couldn't be happier.

Now in my third year of taking Arimidex I began experiencing more severe joint and bone pain as well as daily morning headaches. I changed to a different adjuvant treatment, which after two days caused burning in my esophagus. End of that pill for me, and back onto Arimidex. Everyone is different in how they respond to the various adjuvant treatments. All of adjuvant treatment pills have different side effects. You just have to find the one with the side effects you are willing to tolerate. You may need to switch from one to another until you find the right one for you, and that's okay too.

The best remedy I found for *initial* joint and bone pain caused by the adjuvant treatment is an over-the-counter supplement called Glucosamine with Chondroitin. Now the newest joint supplement is MSM with Glucosamine and Chondroitin. This combination is used to create an advanced joint mobility combo to support joint and mobility comfort. The MSM reportedly provides an organic source of sulfur which is necessary for normal cartilage formation. Glucosamine helps keep collagen supple and Chondroitin provides lubrication to reduce friction and help the joint glide easily.

Research has shown that taking Glucosamine sulfate and Chondroitin sulfate with MSM as a dietary supplement may help reduce bone loss and may also assist in rehabilitating damaged cartilage. It also improves mobility and helps alleviate inflammation. It was a miracle worker for me and many others I know. Also, taking a bath with about two cups of Epsom salts works great for the overall muscle and bone aches you are likely to encounter. Over-the-counter Ibuprofin or brand-name arthritis pain caplets also help relieve joint pain.

After a couple of years of being on an adjuvant treatment pill, many people get to the point where they need to take prescriptive pain medication to function without constant joint and muscle pain due to continuous depletion of estrogen. That does not mean that you will necessarily experience those same side effects. If you think your joint or bone pain may be more severe, you might want to check with your doctor to see if a prescriptive pain medication might be right for you.

Consider also being tested for your bone density to see if you may need something to reverse bone loss. The bone density test is totally painless, and the procedure doesn't take much time at all. The worst part is having to weigh yourself, which by now you should be used to because the doctors weigh you every time you turn around. Many chemos these days cause temporary weight gain of approximately fifteen pounds. So, I just face the opposite direction and tell them not to tell me what my weight is. One day I'll take it off, hopefully.

It is encouraging to know that research has also shown that taking certain prescriptive medications may assist in rejuvenating any bone loss suffered. *However, make sure to ask your doctor if the prescribed medication may cause necrosis (death) of the jawbone.* It has recently been documented that some of the most common restorative bone enhancers cause death of the jawbone.

Although we may think, and hope, that physical activity may be detrimental to the health of our bones and joints, it is not. Physical activity is essential to joint care. It helps your range of motion and keeps bone loss from getting worse. Exercising can simply be stretching your body for ten or fifteen minutes a day. Yoga is also very good and is soothing emotionally; the latest studies support this. However, this is not the time to ridiculously think you are lazy if you are not participating in the exercises you have enjoyed in the past. Your body is under stress and it needs a little TLC. Just allow yourself time to heal. You will progress in your activity participation in your own time.

The Fatigues

Throughout my treatment, which includes continuing with Arimidex, just watching people jog makes me exhausted. We happen to live near a university and across the street from a park. College students jog at all hours of the day. I see people playing volleyball, rollerblading, and playing soccer. I also see the elderly playing doubles in tennis and wonder where in the world they get their energy. But you know what? It's okay. When you are going through treatment, just know that you will be naturally exhausted, especially throughout the beginning treatments. However, the exhaustion lessens as you continue in your treatment, taking all of the medications your doctor prescribes so that your cancer will hopefully never return. Be easy on yourself. You need rest so allow yourself to relax. There will be plenty of time to exercise later.

Sometimes there is the fear that if we change our routine, we will succumb to the breast cancer; so we keep on working until we just about collapse. Although this is understandable, it really is not necessary unless you absolutely have to work. In fact, stress is something we, as breast cancer patients, are to avoid at all costs because it hinders the healing process.

Naively, the morning of my first chemo I was so determined to keep my routine that I made Ahmad drive me right back to work (I can be a little bit obsessive). However, I quickly learned this wasn't such a hot idea. When he drove me to my last appointment that day, I began to feel quite nauseous toward the end. As soon as I got into the car to go home, there, into a bag designated for such a possibility, went my lunch. I quickly learned that I had to take at least four or five days off after my chemo sessions, as those are the days a person usually feels most nauseous. Because of this, many people choose to have chemo treatments on a Friday.

Still insisting I keep my life normal, I went back to work two weeks after my lumpectomy and continued for two months until just before my second chemo, when I got so light-headed that I collapsed when I got home. The next morning I called my office to let them know

I couldn't keep going, and that I had to take a medical leave. They understood and were very kind about it.

I was so relieved to be able to get the rest I so desperately needed. Then one day I was reading the *23rd Psalm,* which most people are familiar with regardless of their religion. However, this day I saw it in a different way. The beginning of it goes like this:

The Lord is my shepherd;
I shall not want.
He maketh me to lie down in green pastures:
He leadeth me by the still waters.
He restoreth my soul...
—*The Bible: Psalm 23*
King James Version

Wow! I thought as I laughed. Sometimes we get so busy with our lives that we do not allow time for rejuvenating ourselves. I could just hear God say, "Now, Joyce, you sit here in this green pasture." And indeed, although the treatment was very difficult on me physically, I finally surrendered to allow my spirit, body and soul to be rejuvenated. If you resist the journey you will be miserable, and you will miss all the good things this trial can do for you spiritually and emotionally.

I would also encourage you to consider going to a nutritional store to talk to a nutritionist regarding the fatigue due to chemo and/or radiation. Ask what vitamins, liquids or capsules they can suggest that might help you. However, before you start taking any vitamins or especially Chinese herbs you will need to consult with your physician to make sure they will not interfere with any of your treatments. I was able to find some vitamins that truly helped me get quite a bit of my energy back.

Chemobrain

Chemobrain is not actually as bad as it sounds. Basically, chemobrain is a loss of memory as well as loss of focus and/or concentration. Those problems are really more irritating than anything else. For example, sometimes I still find myself talking to someone, and for the life of me, I just cannot remember a descriptive word that used to come naturally. So, depending on the person(s) I am talking to, I might admit that I can't remember the darn word and I explain it in simple terms. Then, once the moment is lost, it may or may not come back to me. That can be quite frustrating, but I am still thankful because things could be a lot worse.

Also, due to chemobrain, I often forget how to spell a lot of words. But again, these are solvable irritations, and sometimes I think it is funny. You have to laugh at yourself sometimes. Don't make life so serious. Just remember, the brain is like a muscle. The cells in the brain are also able to rejuvenate themselves. The more you exercise your brain, the stronger and the more precise it will become.

As far as your ability to pay attention or concentrate during and after chemo, it is likely that these problems could be caused not only by chemo but by the medications that must be taken. The depression that usually tags along with the disease, the feelings of being overwhelmed and many other feelings, come along because of this illness. So don't be so hard on yourself. Just remember, this is most often a temporary condition, and this too shall pass.

How in the World do they Make Nipples?

Nipple reconstruction is usually done about six months after a mastectomy with reconstruction. I am extremely happy with the nipple reconstruction we chose. We chose nipple and areola reconstruction using skin that is taken from the bikini line, where the skin appears darker in color once it is placed on the breast. At first the nipple appears quite large, but after six months to a year it reduces to a normal size.

Another way to reconstruct a nipple after a breast has healed from surgery is that a plastic surgeon makes a new nipple and areola from your own breast. The doctor makes an incision in the shape of a star to create the new nipple and then the sides of each of the flaps are raised up so that the middle of the flap poofs up, making it thicken as it advances toward the middle. Once the sides are poofed up they are re-attached from the top of the nipple, making the nipple protrude. Then, once the nipple heals, it can be tattooed a natural color and they can also tattoo the surrounding areola. (It is just my opinion, but I think a nipple is more likely to "live" if you *add* skin to it rather than open the skin and restructure the inside tissue.) I have also heard enough women discuss their disappointment with the cosmetic result of the latter procedure to have formulated this opinion.

About eight months after my bilateral mastectomy, my reconstructive surgeon, Dr. Linda Li, made my areola and nipples with a skin graft taken from my bikini line area. The areola and nipples look so natural that unless they are looked at closely one cannot tell the difference.

There are also other ways of reconstructing nipples depending on the type of reconstructive surgery that you and your doctor choose. The above two methods appear to be the most common, especially with implant reconstruction.

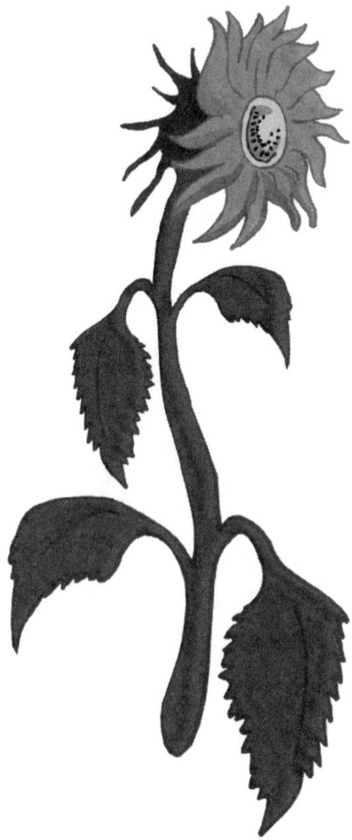

CHAPTER SIX

Life Goes On

Our Little Wedding

Ahmad and I married September 20, 2003, about a year and a half after my first breast cancer treatment. We decided we wanted to have a private wedding, so we made reservations to be married in a beautiful chapel in Las Vegas. We didn't realize it until after we reserved the chapel, but we were actually getting married on the anniversary of our first date! It was such a special day for both of us. We also had a lot of fun in Vegas, plus I won a nice little jackpot. Five weeks later we went to Hawaii for our honeymoon. We both felt we had found our soulmate, and we still feel that way!

Women Who Found Their Soulmate During Breast Cancer

One young woman with whom I am familiar met her husband in the chemo chair. They both were receiving chemo and began to chat. One thing led to another, and they became boyfriend and girlfriend for a couple of years. His cancer went into remission, but hers, unfortunately, continued. He married her while she was in Stage IV because he loved her, regardless.

Another young woman was abandoned by her boyfriend of two years, specifically because she had breast cancer. She was deeply hurt, but several months later she met a very handsome young man in a restaurant while she was wearing her wig. He pursued her despite her reluctance. She finally gave him her phone number. As they talked for hours on the phone, she accidentally mentioned her appointment with her "oncologist." Although he understood, he said nothing of it and made a date with her. When they met on their first date she did not want to be hurt again, so she let him know up front that she had breast cancer. She also told him she had just had a double mastectomy with reconstruction and was bald because of her chemo. He said he didn't care. He liked her for who she was. Soon after that they moved in together. I have lost touch with them, but the point is, there is always hope despite seemingly hopeless circumstances. As long as you are willing to believe in miracles you just might experience one!

Some don't believe in miracles.
They say, "What happens is by chance."
They rush through God's creation
Without a passing glance.
But for those that look and listen
throughout each precious day
They will find the tracks of Angels,
as they move along their way!
— Andie Hellem

If Your Breast Cancer Spreads to the Lymph Nodes or Metastasizes Beyond

Many, many breast cancer women live long happy lives despite the statistics. Just because your breast cancer has spread to the lymph nodes, it doesn't necessarily mean that it will metastasize anywhere else. There are so many advances in breast cancer treatment today that you will be amazed. Even if your breast cancer metastasizes elsewhere in your body, because of the advances in breast cancer, many women still live happily for years afterward. As Abraham Lincoln once said, "Most people are about as happy as they make up their minds to be."

I am acquainted with several Stage IV women. One of them is young, married, and has a young daughter. She still keeps hopeful, despite fighting all odds. She loves to spend as much time as possible in her garden and with her daughter. These are places where she gains her strength.

Another Stage IV woman finally decided she'd had enough chemotherapy. As a matter of fact, she felt like the doctors were "killing her" with too much chemotherapy, so she decided to try alternative medicines instead. I had never seen her look or feel so good.

Don't Quit

When things go wrong, as they sometimes will
When the road you're trudging seems all uphill
When the funds are low and the debts are high
And you want to smile, but you have to sigh
When care is pressing you down a bit
Rest, you must—but don't you quit
Life is queer with its twists and turns
As everyone of us sometimes learns.
And many a failure turns about
When he might have won had he stuck it out
Don't give up, though the pace seems slow
You might succeed with another blow
Success is failure turned inside out,
the silver tint on the clouds of doubt
And you never can tell how close you are,
It may be near when it seems so far
It's when things seem worst,
That you MUST NOT QUIT!

—Author Unknown

Don't Beat Yourself Up

If your breast cancer has spread to the lymph nodes or has metastasized to other parts of your body, it most likely is not because you waited too long to get yourself checked. So don't beat yourself up. Researchers, including my breast surgeon, Dr. Bret Taback, then at the John Wayne Cancer Institute in Santa Monica, California, have found that there are some types of breast cancer that basically spread immediately because they do not have the Breast Cancer Metastasis Suppressor 1 gene (BCMS1).

According to researchers, "It may be several years before a lump appears in the breast after cancer starts. The disease behavior is unpredictable. It may spread quickly into nearby lymph nodes under the arm or stay confined to the breast for a long time." www.jwci.org/AboutCancerBreast/FAQs.htm#l4

In a different study led by Dr. Danny Welch from Pennsylvania State University College of Medicine in Hershey, the authors state, "In a search for genes that prevent breast cancer, a team of researchers noticed that metastasis did not occur when a normal version of a certain chromosome was introduced into breast cancer cells grown in the laboratory. After a search of this chromosome—chromosome 11—they identified the gene as a possible metastasis suppressor gene…(BRMS1, or Breast Cancer Metastasis Supressor 1)."

To test the effects of BRMS1, the researchers studied two groups of mice. One group was implanted with human breast cancer cells that had the gene introduced into the cells, while the other received breast cancer cells without the added gene. In both groups of mice, tumors continued to grow at about the same rate, the investigators report in the *Journal of Cancer Research.*

But metastasis was much less in mice who received the BRMS1, suggesting that when the gene is damaged or mutated, cells are more likely to spread. Mice given a functional copy of the BRMS1 gene had a 50 to 90 percent reduction in tumors in the lymph nodes and lungs compared with other mice, according to this report. While this strategy could never be used to treat breast cancer patients, there is no easy way to put BRMS1 inside cancer cells growing in the body. However, it does shed light on the gene's function.

According to Welch and colleagues, "Since the most lethal attribute of breast cancer cells is their ability to spread and colonize distant sites, understanding the BRMS1 function may help prevent metastasis and improve breast cancer survival…" The authors note that, to date, "only six other genes have been identified that can help suppress cancer metastasis in animal studies." www.wired.com / news / technology / 0,1282,36770,00.html

What are the Risk Factors for Breast Cancer? (So You Can Answer Your Family and Friends)

Most of us who have, or have had, breast cancer, have found that our friends and family are not only concerned about us, but they naturally begin to wonder what their risk factors are for getting breast cancer. Well, just so that you're not at a loss for words when they ask you, whom they now count upon to be the expert, here are some universally known risks for breast cancer:

1. *When did you start your menstrual cycle?*
   Risk increases the earlier a woman starts her menstrual cycle.

2. *When did you give birth to your first child?*
   The later a woman has her first child the greater the risk. When a woman has her first child at age 30 or older she is considered at greater risk. Also, if a woman does not give birth to children at all she is at a higher risk.

3. *How many immediate family members have you had with breast cancer?*
   The more immediate relatives you have had breast cancer, the greater the risk of acquiring it.

4. *What race are you?*
   White women, especially from Northern America, are more likely to get breast cancer than Hispanic, African-American or Asian women.

5. *What is your age?*
   The older we get, the higher our risk.

6. *Have you had any previous biopsies?*
   The more breast biopsies you've had the greater the risk.

7. *Have you ever had a biopsy that was diagnosed as atypical?*

   Doctors use different terms for various atypical biopsies, but if you've had a biopsy that was diagnosed as "atypical" you are at higher risk.

8. *Have you had a lot of red meat and high-fat dairy products in your diet?*
   Animal fat, especially from red meat and high-fat dairy products, increases the risk of breast cancer.

8. *How dense are your breasts?*
   The denser the breasts the greater the risk for breast cancer.

9. *Did you go through menopause at a late age?*
   Late menopause can be a risk factor for breast cancer because of the amount of estrogen your body continues to receive.

Regardless of the answers that your family and friends give to these questions, as soon as they find out you have breast cancer most of them will run out and get a mammogram as soon as possible! Now that's a good thing.

Also, if your friends or family would like to take a Breast Cancer Risk Test, you can go to www.halls.md/breast/risk.htm

Laugh Yourself Better

Many of us know the story of Norman Cousins who, over thirty years ago, overcame a crippling terminal illness by watching and laughing at old comedies. Laughter truly does have a natural biological healing effect. According to the LaRoche and the American Cancer Society, laughter boosts the immune system by increasing T-cell count. It also boosts your immune system by increasing other killer cell production. White blood cell activity is increased. Further, laughing can increase the production of elemental immune system cells and gamma-interferon, which is believed to fight cancer.

In addition, according to experts, laughter increases blood circulation, stabilizes blood pressure, and provides increased oxygen supply to muscles, leading to reduced tension. It also facilitates digestion and massages our inner organs, giving us a sense of well-being. Laughter also helps us sleep well. There are now hospitals and cancer support groups all over the nation that are incorporating laughter into their rehabilitation. They have provided special rooms with comedic materials and television comedy to encourage people to laugh.

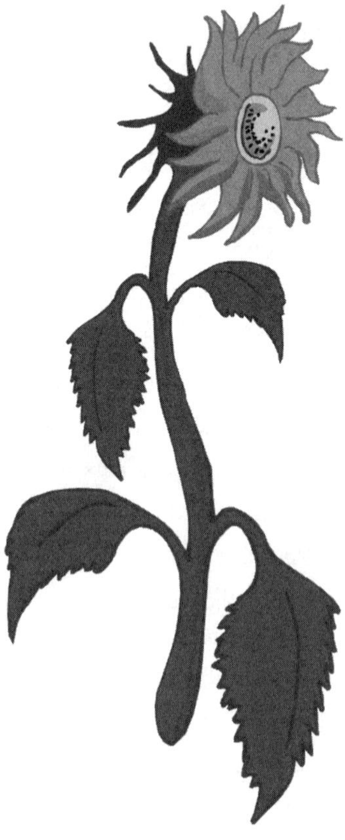

Summary

Breast cancer is no longer an automatic death sentence. Instead, allow this trial to make you into a better person. Most people have no idea the gifts that await them when they are given a trial. Immediately they begin to fear the worst. In fact, like me, God can use this situation to bring you closer to Him. He can also use it to bring others closer to you. In your darkest hours, if you reach out, you have no idea the blessings that will come your way.

—Joyce Giannini

FOR MORE INFORMATION, PLEASE CONTACT:

Atlas Books

P.O. Box 388

Ashland, OH 44805

Tel: 1 (800) 266-5564

Fax: 1 (419) 281-6883

www.atlasbooks.com

We invite you to visit our website:

www.BreastCancerHopeBook.com

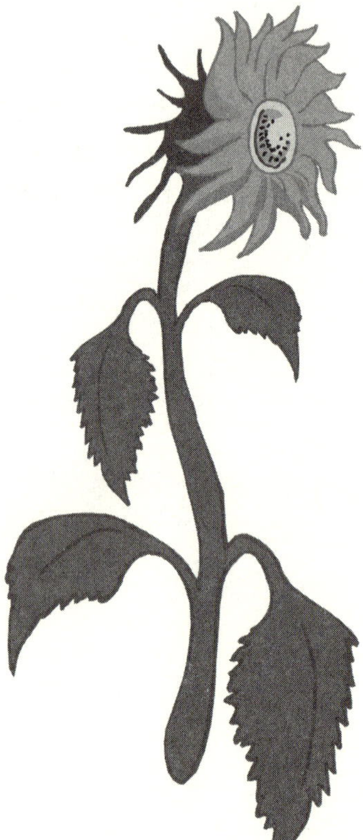